YOUR
FAMILY
DOCTOR
ASTHMA

YOUR FAMILY DOCTOR

ASTHMA

Understanding Asthma • Avoiding Allergies • Proper Use of Inhalers

DR VINOD WADHWA

wisdom
tree

© Dr Vinod Wadhwa, 2006

ISBN 81-8328-033-1

Published by

Wisdom Tree
4779/23 Ansari Road
Darya Ganj, New Delhi-110002
Ph.: 23247966/67/68

Published by Shobit Arya for Wisdom Tree; *edited by* Manju Gupta; *designed by* Kamal P. Jammual; *typeset at* Icon Printographics, New Delhi-110018 and *printed at* Print Perfect, New Delhi-110064

"Don't look at the low points in your life as defeats, but as opportunities to make progress."

These lines are particularly true for asthmatics as there are low points when one has an acute attack of asthma, fortunately followed by periods of remission. So let the spirit soar as tough times lead to a healthy tomorrow.

This book is dedicated to all men and women who strive to give us a healthy, pollution-free planet.

Contents

Preface

Over the years, a group of environmentalists have been crying hoarse over the degradation of our planet's environment. No wonder the cases of respiratory disorders are on the increase. This small work explains the concepts of allergy and bronchial asthma in concise. This would be handy for asthmatics and their well-wishers.

Acknowledgements

You can do a thing quite well by yourself but you can do it a lot better with help from others. My acknowledgements to Dr Dietrich Nolte, M.D. whose book, *Speaking of Asthma* encouraged me to write about asthma. My gratitude to Dr O.P. Jaggi for his inspiring book, *Asthma and Allergies*.

Introduction

The term 'asthma' is about 2,500-years old, though the disease itself must be as old as the human race itself. When man started recording events, then his health- and disease-related issues came to be understood. The great Greek doctor, Hippocrates, studied this disease which caused coughing, wheezing and breathlessness. He also noted episodes of acute breathlessness and periods when there was no difficulty in breathing. He named this disease as 'asthma'.

Asthma today is described as a disease which shows reversible obstruction of the chest passages accompanied by attacks of breathlessness and followed by periods which are symptom-free.

This disease knows no geographical or racial barriers or boundaries. There could be differences in rates of incidence but it has a worldwide

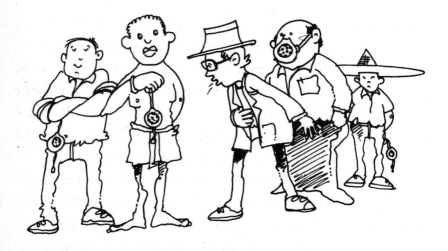

distribution, so much so that native races and tribes living in deep forests with almost no contact with the developed world, are also known to suffer from it. Thus, it is neither a new disease nor a disease inflicted upon humans because of urbanisation or industrialisation.

> **There are an estimated 9 million asthmatics worldwide. Nearly 2–7 per cent of the general population could be suffering from bronchial asthma.**

The incidence of asthma in the general population is difficult to assess because there are no fixed parameters for diagnosis and also because asthmatics do not always suffer from breathlessness bouts. No wonder 2–7 per cent of our population is said to be suffering from bronchial asthma. Age- and sex-specific indices throw an interesting fact. Among children, twice as many boys as girls suffer from asthma but during adulthood, one-and-a-half times more women compared to men suffer from asthma. How and why this change comes up is a subject of speculation, till research throws some concrete evidence.

The atmosphere, which we usually take for granted, is a source of energy for almost all organisms. The air that we breathe in (inhale) through our nostrils enters our lungs where it binds to the haemoglobin in our red blood cells (erythrocytes) to generate oxyhaemoglobin. The oxyhaemoglobin reaches all parts of the body through the blood where the tissues are hungry for energy. Oxygen separates from its haemoglobin carrier and carbon dioxide from the tissues now uses this haemoglobin for transportation. The oxygen thus made available is thankfully used by the cells for energy.

Strange as it may sound, this life-giving air could be the cause of misery for human beings. Dust, pollen, infection-causing organisms like bacteria, viruses and fungal spores could enter our body with air and befool the body's defence mechanism, thereby causing respiratory diseases. I often marvel at God's plan of providing a great defence mechanism to an organism and at the same time encouraging other organisms to develop counter mechanisms. Only He knows best!!

Considering the vagaries of Nature and our earth's ever-changing environment, God created a respiratory system which could easily take on all these variations.

The nostrils have the triple job of heating or cooling the air, filtering off the harmful pollutants and microorganisms from the air and humidifying it as it enters the body. The nostrils thus work as the first barrier in the fight against the dust, pollutants and the potential disease-

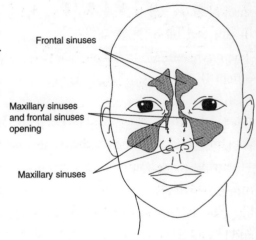

causing microorganisms. The lining in the nostrils has fine hair-like projections called 'cilia' which trap dust and the invading organisms. This lining is all the time bathed in a secretion called 'mucus' which prevents the tissues from drying and also helps to dampen the inhaled air. This mucus also traps microorganisms, harmful gases and

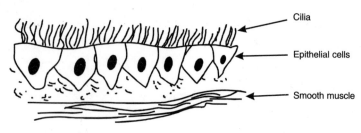

Cilia

Epithelial cells

Smooth muscle

Lining of cells with cilia

chemicals, which, if allowed to enter the lungs, could induce bouts of coughing and swelling of the lung tissues with dire consequences. Thus, this great design of the Lord makes a human nose a great sentry to the portals of the respiratory system.

The air now moves into the windpipe and then enters the lungs. The large airways divide and subdivide many times, with the subdivisions becoming narrower and narrower. All these tubes are lined by the same kind of surface epithelium as the nostrils. The mucus and the cilia are present here also to assist in the respiratory functioning.

Respiration or breathing has two physical components —

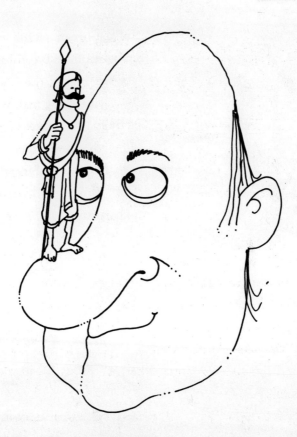

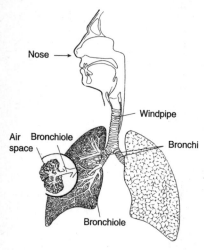

Lungs with the bronchial tree

inhalation or taking in of air and exhalation or breathing out of air. As we inhale, the volume of the lungs increases mainly due to the activity of the muscular diaphragm. Then the chest returns to its original size, thereby pushing the air out of the lungs. This constitutes exhalation.

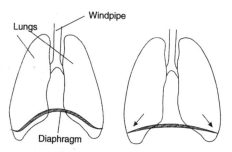

Expiration: Breathing out   Inspiration: Breathing in

Mucus, the sticky sentry

The entire airway is covered by a very thin layer of mucus. This mucus plays the role of trapping toxic gases and the invading microorganisms. It also tends to hydrate the air that enters the lungs with each inhalation.

CHAPTER ONE

What is asthma?

When we say that a person has asthma, it means that the person has sensitive lungs or sensitive bronchi. The bronchi are tubes that convey the air we breathe from the nose and windpipe to the lungs. They are like pipes made of smooth muscle.

Like all muscles in the body, these muscle cells contract when stimulated. Therefore, these tubes are able to vary their diameter, thus allowing more (or less) air to flow in and out of the lungs as needed at various times.

Unfortunately in a person who has asthma, these air passages are overly sensitive to certain stimuli referred to as allergens or substances present in the air we breathe; substances that get into the body through food or through the skin; and sometimes even emotional stimuli. When exposed to these stimuli, the air tubes suddenly become narrow, making it difficult for air to flow into the lungs. The result is difficulty in breathing, with concomitant wheezing and air hunger.

Sudden and repeated episodes of shortness of breath with 'wheezing' sound (heard more often on breathing out) convey that the person suffers from asthma. This is associated with a feeling of tightness or heaviness in the chest followed by an irritating cough which is usually dry. At times, a small amount of mucus or phlegm is released (expectorate). The phlegm becomes copious and yellowish or greenish after an infection sets in. What frightens a lot of patients is the blackish, soot-like excrustation on the phlegm which incidentally is nothing but the pollutants that were inhaled. This just shows the level of pollution and the extent of fossil fuel use. There is a silver lining to all this and this is the reversible nature of the asthmatic attacks. Bronchial asthma is a reversible and temporary disease and once an acute attack is over, the patient's respiratory system is restored back to its normal status.

> There are close to 300 million alveoli or air sacs in human lungs. These alveoli are tiny air sacs with 0.3 mm diameter. These constitute the site of air exchange through the blood. If the alveoli are opened up, they could easily be as large as four badminton courts.

Asthma could be broadly classified into *extrinsic asthma* (allergic asthma) and *intrinsic asthma*. Often, most people think asthma and allergy are synonymous. Let's discuss the two terms in detail as the term 'allergy' needs to be understood to get the hang of the term 'asthma'.

Actually, simply put, 'allergy' means 'to react differently'; it is the reaction of a person to something to which most people would not react. Let me elaborate upon this with the example of pollen. At most times of the year, all sorts of pollen are present in the air in considerable numbers. All of us keep inhaling them throughout the day, without

---

Warning signs

The American Academy of Paediatrics has given a list of warning signs that tell you an asthma attack is imminent:

- **Breathing is difficult and faster than usual.**
- **Wheezing, coughing and shortness of breath.**
- **Problem in breathing may affect speech.**
- **Skin colour may become paler than usual.**
- **A decrease in the level of awareness.**
- **When drawing in of the muscles between the ribs becomes necessary to breathe.**

showing any evidence of any problem but there are some people (10-15 per cent of our population) who show "altered reaction to this specific substance". They could suffer from sneezing, running nose, burning and stinging in the eyes and at times, cough accompanied by difficulty in breathing and wheezing. All these signs indicate altered sensitivity to a substance which others would not react to.

Now, that the concept of the term 'allergy' is clear, let us find out how it is caused. In allergic people, this pollen works like an allergen or antigen which, on exposure, induces the production of a specific protein called 'antibody' or reagin. This invading allergen meets the antibody to bring about an antigen–antibody reaction. If this occurs on a cell called the 'mast cell', it sets off instability of the cell membrane which eventually ruptures to liberate a veritable chemical weaponry of sorts. Chemicals like histamine, serotonin and SRS (slow-reacting substances), to name a few, are thus released from the mast cells causing the common physical manifestations of allergic reaction, viz. the weal-and-flare reaction. These could cause:

- Swelling, redness, itching of the skin as seen in urticaria.

- Secretion of a clear, watery fluid from the lining of the nose as seen in allergic rhinitis.
- Constriction or spasm in the muscles of the airways of lungs as seen in asthma. The first two reactions also occur in the airways, i.e. swelling and mucus secretion to cause symptoms of cough and wheezing.

Thus, allergy could have different manifestations in different individuals and may run in families with the allergic predisposition. Allergies are highly unpredictable, appearing and disappearing suddenly but there is now a corpus of researchers which believes that people with an allergic manifestation or predisposition could show different allergic symptoms at different times or phases of life. Let's clarify this statement.

Certain children during infancy show redness and swelling of the skin which is itchy. These lesions are seen in the flexures (body folds) like the elbow, the back of the knees, the neck and occasionally, the groin. This allergic eczema disappears as dramatically as it appears (with usually the last doctor getting the benefit of doubt of having managed to cure the child). Only Nature knows best. No sooner does the allergy disappear, the young child could develop bouts of running nose, sneezing, red and itchy eyes in a particular season. If the cold lasts longer, the child would then become breathless and wheezing would develop. This illustrates that some people are born with a predisposition to allergies. Furthermore, there are families which show a greater tendency towards allergic manifestation, though the spectrum could be different in different family members.

> **Sinusitis, an inflammation of the perinasal sinuses, could cause bronchial asthma. Nasal polyps are also incriminated similarly. Therefore, one could try and manage perinasal sinusitis as early as possible.**

Common allergens

Though human beings could be allergic to almost anything under the sun or for that matter, even the sun itself at times, there are certain things which could be put under the category of common allergens. To enumerate, these are:

- Pollen
- House dust
- Moulds
- Pets, both animals and birds
- Pollutants

Pollen: Much has been written about this extremely small yet major troublemaker. It has been blamed as the commonest cause of both allergic rhinitis and bronchial asthma. Pollen is the fine dust produced by flowers and this dust is carried over long distances by air, insects, water, etc. It is usually the lighter or the smaller pollen which is carried by the wind and could cause problems miles away from where it originates. As most plants have a particular flowering season, one can predict the pollen that is most likely to cause a problem at a particular time of the year. It is best to avoid an area which abounds in pollen during the pollen calendar a person is allergic to and in case that is not possible, it is best to start on medicines early.

One could be allergic to a single pollen species or show allergy to many different species of pollen. Some nasal filters are available in the market with simple (crude, if I may say so) gadgets which one could auto-fit into the nostrils and remove at will. One does see encouraging results with this simple gadget.

House dust: How very clean you might think your house to be, you cannot banish dust from your dwelling. It is all pervasive. Dust is actually a cocktail of particles of different sizes, shapes and composition. Pungent items like chillies or pepper could cause a bout of sneezing in anyone, but house dust can cause this reaction only among those who are allergy-prone. Often you may have experienced a bout after cleaning old books or clothes which could be covered with a layer of dust. What really causes allergy is something which you can hardly smell or see. You can smell tobacco or burning cigarette paper, chemicals from aerosols and moth balls or the smell of fat escaping from the frying pan. It is now known that the real cause of trouble is a small, little villain called the 'dust mite'. It is a small insect, about one-third of a millimetre in size and it could happily stay on human skin when the old, dead cells from the skin are shed. This little rascal accompanies the cells. It could stay for days on the furnishings as dust till the dust is disturbed. The strange habit of dusting furniture and furnishings violently makes this dust mite airborne and it could easily gain entry into the human body through the nose. Once it does so, it sets up an allergic reaction. This mite thrives best in high-moisture and high-temperature climates. Hot and dry climates therefore are usually safer for people with allergy to house dust. More and more insects, especially cockroaches and their sheddings are now being researched as the likely cause for allergic reactions related to house dust. Though difficult, one can always make an effort to avoid contact with house dust. The following list of do's and don'ts would be in order:

- Always vacuum clean the floor, furnishings, etc. and follow it up with wet mopping of the floor.
- Use a chimney or an exhaust fan in the kitchen.

- Avoid aerosols, burning of incense sticks, etc. indoors.
- Avoid cutflowers indoors.
- Avoid, if possible, the use of woollen carpets or if in use, vacuum clean these regularly.
- Brush pets outdoors.
- Regular pest control should be done.
- Make sure the rooms get enough sunshine and proper ventilation.

Moulds: Moulds or fungi are almost always present in the air around us. Not all fungi are potentially harmful; in fact, only a few have made the entire clan suspect. Fungi and their spores are often found floating in air and can enter our respiratory system. Despite all protection, some fungal spores do reach the airways and cause asthma among the allergy-prone. Basements, which are usually dark and damp with poor ventilation, are known to harbour plenty of fungal spores. Aircon-ditioners are notorious in allowing fungi a permanent abode. Some fungi can cause allergies while other fungi are potentially disease-causing, especially in immuno-compromised patients. Lawns, potted plants, rotting vegetable matter and animal dander are all great hosts and could have a high mould population in geographical areas with high rainfall and poor sunshine.

An interesting finding is that most people who are allergic to moulds are also allergic to quite a few pollen species and vice versa, making it difficult to diagnose as to what is the specific allergen.

Pets: Pets, though most often a source of joy, could at times be a source of allergy and asthma. Most people who love pets refuse to see the logic in this statement and continue to wheeze while looking for alternative treatments. Some people are allergic to animal hair and dander while others are allergic to the dried saliva of animals and to bird feathers. Cats, dogs, horses and almost all birds could cause allergies. The only way to confirm an allergy to pets is to either relocate the pet for some time or, if possible, to move out of your house but stay in close vicinity. If your separation relieves you of the allergy, then the diagnosis is confirmed and the treatment is obvious — a total fracture of man-animal bond. You could be gracious enough to gift your pet to a person who is not inclined as you are to asthma and could

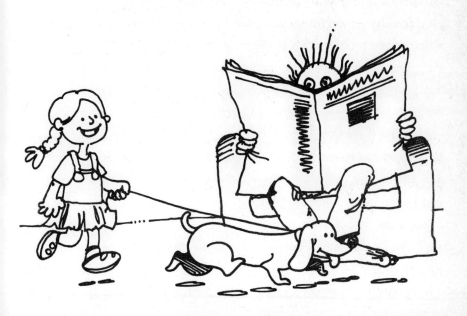

enjoy the company of the pet without suffering. A few tears in compensation for years of misery with a pet around!

Heredity vs environment: Not long ago, asthma was considered a hereditary problem. Most clinicians do not want to be committal, thus the hereditary vs environment debate continues and is gathering more support. To support the hereditary theory is the fact that identical twins show a greater evidence of asthma, but this could also mean that the common environment of the twins is implicated. The same macro and micro environment could be the cause for such findings. After all the debate, one point emerges clearly and that is, a certain degree of role is played by heredity, with the environment contributing the triggering factors. Despite the fact that now the acceptance of hereditary causative factors is widespread, we still do not know how the allergic process would manifest in the progeny. To clarify, a child might suffer from infantile eczema, yet another child from the same family may show signs of hay fever or bronchial asthma.

No less confusing is another cause that has long been implicated and it is the psychosomatic factor. There have been many studies and research on the role of the psyche in possible acute exacerbations of asthma but, as the basic cause for asthma, psyche is not held responsible. Emotional distress or stress could possibly precipitate an asthmatic attack in a person with an allergic predisposition. The role of meditation and relaxation techniques therefore cannot be overemphasised.

Another cause-effect relationship that has been implicated is the allergy-infection-allergy cycle. An indepth study in children has shown a correlation. After a seasonal cold or cough, usually caused by viruses, children might start showing evidence of bronchial asthma. These attacks are rare and usually disappear with appropriate management of the infection with bronchodilators. At the same time, children suffering from bronchial asthma have a lot of mucus or phlegm which attracts a range of viruses and bacteria. These disease-causing microorganisms flourish in this mucus media and cause recurrent infections. Most of the times, initial asthmatic attacks would be a passing phase, with the patient recovering quickly and completely. Though this should ring an alarm bell for the attending physician, it then becomes his duty to advise the patient to take trivial infections also very seriously. Repeated infections increase the chances of prolonged phases of wheezing and breathlessness. This cascading effect causes a lot of misery to young children. In such dire conditions, one needs to manage both problems in one go, rather than meeting each challenge individually.

Another influencing factor is the house architecture and place of residence. People with asthma are usually better off in dry places as compared to humid, moist places or seashores. The level of pollen and automobile discharge are also very important factors. Most weather reports talk about the level of suspended impurities in the atmosphere. Toxic gases (usually emanating from burning of fossil fuels) also cause asthma and at times, permanent damage to the respiratory system.

CHAPTER TWO

Do you have asthma?

Tools of diagnosis

Attacks of asthma are usually so dramatic and so sudden that anybody who has seen or, God forbid, experienced one such episode, would identify it easily. The patient is fine one minute and suddenly, he or she could have a bout of dry cough initially, followed by an intense difficulty in breathing. Most attacks occur after midnight, usually around 2 a.m. or 3 a.m. Lots of asthmatics tend to start coughing at around this time and then expectorate some tenacious phlegm before

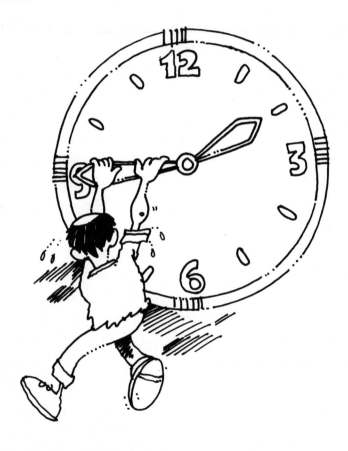

getting some relief. As the cough and breathless spell starts, a panic reaction begins and causes more and more muscular exertion and discomfort. At this point of time, it is extremely important to take sustained-release theophylline to avoid the 2 a.m. or 3 a.m.-syndrome, particularly if panic takes the better of an asthmatic patient. At the beginning of the attack, the symptoms get magnified and cause great trouble to the patient and the family. Attacks could get precipitated by dust, tobacco, smoke or insecticide sprays. Paints, varnishes and aerosols could also trigger off an attack. Physical exertion, especially in cold weather, is known to bring about acute asthmatic attacks.

What happens in an acute attack?

When the patient suffers from an acute attack, the chest is most noisy and, believe me, it produces the most astounding sounds. There could be whistling, wheezing sounds and high-pitched sonorous sounds. The stethoscope helps to diagnose and in technical jargon these sounds are clubbed under the term 'rhonchi'. During an acute attack, with release of all the chemicals we discussed earlier on, there is swelling and

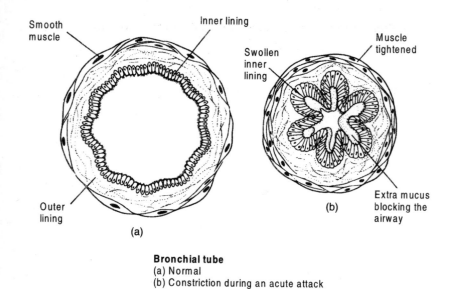

Bronchial tube
(a) Normal
(b) Constriction during an acute attack

increased mucus production in the chest airways. Also, the smooth muscles which line these passages tend to contract, thus decreasing the lumen of these passages. As a result, when air during expiration is pushed out through the narrow passages, a typical sound is produced. Air under pressure helps to dislodge thick, tenacious mucus secretions which tend to rattle and add to the spectrum of the sounds produced. All these sounds make the chest really noisy. All this could last from minutes to days. As the attack abates, the chest sounds return to normal and all the secretions get cleared. At this point of time, if a physician listens to or auscultates the chest, he might be fooled altogether. Thus, in between the acute attacks, the chest is pretty much normal with no extra sounds being produced.

Pulmonary function test is a very simple procedure. In this, the patient is made to breathe in and then breathe out into a mouthpiece. The volume of air pushed out is called the 'vital capacity'. This index was considered important earlier but now a new parameter, called FEV or Forced Expiratory Volume in one second, is in vogue. In this, we find out the volume of air expelled in the first second of expiration. This gives us more information about the lung function and restriction in lung capacity or in lung function. Simple, convenient and handy devices are now available for use at home by patients to assess the severity of the symptoms at any point of time. This helps the patient to regulate his drug dosage more effectively and intelligently.

More sophisticated instruments called 'plethysmographs' are available.

Hyperventilation syndrome is a strange condition, seen usually in young, anxious women. These women under stress tend to breathe rapidly and deeply. Slowly and gradually they cannot recover from this cycle. Deeper breaths mean exhaling more and more of CO_2 (carbon dioxide), thus showing reduced CO_2 levels in blood leading to spasms in the hands and feet. Such people are made to breathe into and out of a brown bag to increase the CO_2 in inhaled air.

Sputum studies

Sputum is a response of the cells which produce mucus and line the bronchial tree and the nostrils to some allergen or irritating pollutant.

Mucus is produced in considerable amounts. Most asthmatics complain of cough with expectoration, especially in the early morning hours. On microscopic examination, this sputum is full of eosinophils (cells seen in blood as a component of white blood cell series) which indicate an allergic response. Usually, an asthmatic produces whitish, clear, foamy or frothy mucoid sputum which could become thick and lumpy with a distinct yellowish, greenish hue. This is called 'purulent' and indicates the urgent need of an antibiotic to clear the infection. The cause-and-effect theory of infection and asthma has already been discussed and the urgent need to manage bronchial infection is well understood.

Allergy testing: yes or no?

As discussed, asthma and allergies might or might not be related. In cases where an allergic correlation is established, allergy testing is imperative to try and nail the offending allergen. Allergens are more easily identified in young asthmatics. All allergy tests use skin as the testing ground. Skin allergy becomes obvious and can be seen without the help of any aid. Skin testing is safer as the allergen does not enter the body. Thus, the obvious choice for allergy testing is the skin. Allergy testing can be done by:

- *Rubbing*: The suspected allergen is rubbed on the skin surface.
- *Prick test*: This is done usually when the pollen is suspected as the allergen. A drop of pollen solution is put on the lower arm and the skin underneath is punctured. It is definitely not the most pleasant of tests, but the reward is satisfying. An allergy is proved if the test area becomes red, swollen and itchy within 10 to 20 minutes.
- *Intradermal test*: In this, a large number of solutions are injected in the skin, usually of the back. This does definitely test the patient's patience as a number of sites are injected, but it is worth a try, especially in intractable cases.

All these tests are fine but to wrap up the diagnosis and the line of treatment, one needs to know much more about the patient. To confirm if the allergic testing has thrown up the right allergen, one needs to undergo what is called a *provocative test*. In this, the patient is exposed to the positive tested allergen in a solution form right into the respiratory system. If the patient starts coughing and becomes breathless, then one has hit the nail on the head. Of course, one must have all the facilities to manage the asthmatic attack just in case it gets out of control.

With greater knowledge and information at our disposal, we can now ascertain the allergen's role by going in for testing the production of antibodies to the specific antigen in blood. These tests are not employed very often because of their prohibitive costs. Who knows what the future has in its womb? The day is not far when these tests would become commonplace and help us mitigate the sorrow of asthmatics.

CHAPTER THREE

Patient, heal thyself

Before you think of running to the chest specialist with your wheeze, you must get your questions ready. You need to discuss with him as to what all you can do to prevent acute asthmatic bouts. Simple precautions and care could help you out. One must first try and understand that this disease can be controlled and managed with care. Once you have zeroed down on the allergen, you could take simple measures to avoid contact with the allergen. For example, if you are allergic to cats or cigarette smoke, it would be sensible to keep away from cats and people who smoke. However, avoiding people and things that offend you is easier said than done! If it is pollen, one can avoid contact by staying indoors on heavy pollen days. Though, if dust is your enemy, it is quite a daunting task to avoid contact with the notorious, ubiquitous house-dust mite. One should get the house vacuum-cleaned, or get the house dust on window sills, etc. cleaned. Wet mopping of bare floors, regular cleaning of furnishings, etc. would be of great help. People allergic to animals need not nurse thoughts of owning pets. Feather-filled mattresses and pillows need to be gifted away without remorse. Walls with damp patches need to be scraped and repainted after drying. Moulds and mildew are common offenders. The importance of good ventilation with bright sunny rooms and effective air exchanges needs to be understood. Woollen blankets, caps and mufflers could also cause bronchial allergy. If one is exposed to any of these, it would be best to take a bronchodilator inhaler. If one can foresee a possible exposure to some allergen, a preventive inhalation would be in order.

Asthmatics, when suffering from respiratory infections, undergo a worsening of their symptoms. Thus, an effort to prevent infections should be made honestly. Bacterial infections are managed faster and better, thanks to a host of patient-friendly, effective antibiotics. Viral infections are still a challenge, especially for people with debilitated immune status. Flu shots are now advised yearly to all people having bronchial asthma as it does cut down on hospital admissions of asthma cases because of complications.

Certain occupations could definitely cause or precipitate asthmatic attacks. People with allergic chest predisposition need to avoid occupations which expose them to dust, chemicals, agricultural products and fibres, etc. I have an interesting case to illustrate occupational hazards. I had a patient who was a mason by profession. He had recurrent bouts of acute asthma. He went to his hometown for a while, where a well-wisher took him to some quack. Once away from his professional setup, his condition improved and he had no attack for almost seven to eight months. He returned and met me with tall claims of the quack's medicines. I did not discourage him by explaining the whole story but the day he went back to his work, he again had an acute attack. He was back with me the next day. The poor man was speechless and, of course, breathless at the same time. After months of coaxing, he quit his urban profession and went back to his village where he was doing well but the urban lifestyle called him back and he is now working in a security setup and stays indoors. He often comes back to thank me for the advice and says that asthma is a forgotten story now.

Asthma and pregnancy

Pregnant women with a history of asthma usually show a little increase in symptoms in the first trimester. Generally the next two trimesters are more comfortable because of increase in production of cortisone. So, asthmatic women can go ahead with plans for pregnancy.

CHAPTER FOUR

Role of exercise in asthma

When an asthmatic is relatively symptom-free, he can do moderate physical exercise. Some people tend to develop asthma on exercise, which is simply termed as 'exercise asthma'. Such a condition should signal caution and active sports should not be a serious interest for such people. At the other end of the spectrum, some other asthmatics have no increase in symptoms on exercise. For such individuals, a sport of their choice can be indulged in. However, a word of caution — keep inhalers handy while busy in physical exercise.

Also, ambient temperature should not be very low as low temperatures induce acute asthmatic attacks.

During an acute asthmatic episode, because of severe resistance to the bronchial airways, the patient has to use his accessory muscles to breathe. As a result, he starts to put a lot of strain on his upper chest and neck. As attacks become more frequent, this becomes his habit. Later, even during an attack-free phase, he keeps his muscles in a contracted or tense position, thereby causing his neck and upper chest to take up a classical asthmatic posture. Exercises to help relax the upper chest muscles and to retrain the patient to breathe deeper are of paramount importance. Also, the role of the muscular diaphragm in breathing has to be relearnt by the asthmatic.

The first step is to teach the person the right way to breathe. 'Breathing in' remains same but 'breathing out' is more relaxed and slower. The use of abdominal muscles and the diaphragm has to be stressed. As easy way is to ask the patient to push out the abdomen while breathing, thus learning to reuse the diaphragm. It is also believed that asthmatics during an attack become very anxious. This could be a fallout of a basic anxiety neurosis of the asthmatic coupled with a feeling that he or she is fighting for oxygen, causing him or her to tense up his muscles. Thus, it is imperative to teach the asthmatic to relax his entire body. All the muscles in such patients need individual attention. A whole lot of exercises have been devised for relaxing the high tone in the muscles of the neck, the shoulders, the upper chest and the upper arms.

After years and years of teaching these exercises, one comes to the following conclusion — the most basic need is a state of mental relaxation and everything soon follows. If one is in a state of mental relaxation, the brain does send a message to all the skeletal muscles to relax. For this, I always recommend *shavasana* (the posture of the dead body) to be practiced by all asthmatics, especially during the attack-free periods. The physical element of this *asana* is simple to achieve but it is the higher element of mental relaxation which needs time to master. In this yogic *asana*, one lies down on one's back, with the arms by the sides. Try and relax the entire body and now concentrate on your breathing. I advocate a little variation with a little check on

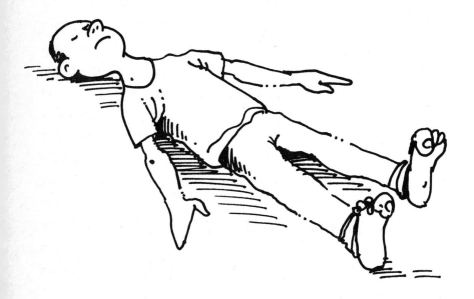

your 'breathing in and breathing out' ratio. Breathing out or expiration should be slow and long in the ratio of 3:2 at the beginning of this relaxation technique. Now start to think of a good, happy event or a beautiful place you want to revisit. You could try to smell the flowers that you are seeing in your mind's eyes or even prepare to hear the sound of flowing water. This is far easier than you think. Lots of yoga instructors tell you to concentrate on the process of breathing in and feeling the air go through the entire body, but I have never been able to achieve this abstract sensation. Possibly one needs to be in a higher state of consciousness about the body. Therefore, I prefer to concentrate on thoughts about beautiful green hills and fragrant meadows. As this happens, the breathing out becomes even more prolonged as you start to breathe slower and deeper. As your mind relaxes, your muscles follow. This is a great technique to learn to relax mentally and physically. A few minutes in the morning, specially on an empty stomach, should help most asthmatics.

There are certain exercises that one can do during an acute attack which would bring about relaxation of the neck and the upper chest.

If one is at home when the attack occurs, one can lie in a semi-reclining position with the head propped up on a couple of pillows. In case a bed is not available, one could sit with the elbows on the knees or on a table. Try and breathe in and then very slowly, breathe out. Try to relax physically and mentally. Do not panic as panic increases the muscle tone, which in turn increases the asthmatic symptoms.

If you are outdoors, you could do this exercise in the standing position with the back resting against a wall or a pole. Once a comfortable posture has been achieved, try and relax your muscles of the neck, shoulders and the upper arms and do not clench your jaw or tighten your fists as this increases your muscle tone. Now try and breathe, using your diaphragm. Raise your abdomen and breathe out very slowly. Do not open your mouth while breathing in because, remember, the nostrils moisten and clear the air before it enters the lungs and this the mouth cannot do. The air being taken in through the mouth hits the pharynx or the back of the throat, causing dryness of the mouth and a sudden bout of coughing. Coughing would aggravate your breathlessness, thereby leading to more panic and starting the cough-wheeze-stress-wheeze cycle.

CHAPTER FIVE

Medicines in asthma

The treatment of asthma actually is the treatment of:
- Acute asthmatic attack (which is easy).
- Asthma or the cause of asthma (which is the real test facing us).

During an acute attack, narrowing of the respiratory passages has to be reverted. Not only this, the narrowing is also accompanied by swelling or oedema of the walls of the bronchial tree with a manifold increase in mucus secretion. This mucus secretion could become thick and tenacious, at the same time encouraging respiratory infections to flourish. Thus, if an acute attack continues for long, the threat of secondary infection has to be taken into consideration. Before I go into the details of the treatment, I would like to dwell on the controversial subject of hyposensitisation.

Hyposensitisation or immunotherapy

In case your asthma is allergic in nature and once you have zeroed down to the pollen that causes allergy, you can go ahead with hyposensitisation or immunotherapy. In this test, the physician prepares a very weak solution (1 in 5,000 dilution) of the allergens to which

> **Drugs called betablockers, which are used to treat hypertension, could cause constriction of the airways, thereby causing bronchial asthma. All of you who are hypertensive with bronchial asthma should avoid betablockers.**

the patient reacts. This solution is then injected into the skin twice a week and one can start with a dose for 0.1 ml which can be increased to a dose of 0.9 ml. Once you are through with this schedule without showing any sign of reaction or allergy, then the strength of the solution can be increased, say, 1 in 500 dilution. Again, one could start with 0.1 ml dose and increase it weekly by 0.1 ml dose till you give a 0.9 ml dose. If everything seems okay, the physician could increase the strength of the solution (1 in 50 dilution) and start injecting all over again.

Results have been variable and physicians are very strongly divided on this issue. Most younger doctors would rather go in for immunoglobulins therapy rather than for this difficult taxing course of subcutaneous injections. The mode of action is still being researched. There are now newer solutions which work for longer periods of time but this is also under scrutiny. Certain people show a reddish swelling in response to the injections, but others could show intense reaction.

I would like to cite a case which makes me shudder even after a good 15 years. A youngish gentleman had been coming to me for these injections. I had just about started to practice independently. As he had taken a good seven to eight injections, he became confident that there could be no problem. With great difficulty, we would make him wait for about 15 minutes after the injection, as stipulated. One day, he decided that enough was enough and physicians were always so fussy that they tend to be real spoilsports. He sauntered out after a couple of minutes of the injection. Fortunately for him, he went to the drug store a few shops down the road. Standing at the drug store, he started to wheeze and then to gasp. The chemist came running to me and I rushed with my bag and my little experience to the site. Believe me, I have never poked in so many injections that I poked into him. Finally, after I had given him two shots of the steroid Decadron, that he said he had started to feel better. I'm sure I could have myself done with a steroid shot to get me out of the shock. A group of onlookers had gathered as if it was a demonstration of sorts. After the whole episode, I decided never to try this form of treatment on anyone and I'm glad I have stuck to my decision. The memory of those few horrific minutes still gives me goose pimples.

Another aspect why hyposensitisation as a form of treatment is on its way out is because asthma in most adults is not allergic. It therefore, has a restricted role as a first-line treatment for asthma, especially in adults.

CHAPTER SIX

Allergic asthma — treatment

As discussed earlier, bronchial asthma could be allergic in nature; in such cases one needs to:

- Avoid contact with the allergens.
- Stabilise the mast cell membrane to block all the chemicals which cause swelling and oedema of the bronchial passages.

We know of certain chemicals that block the rupture of mast cells and thus help in preventing an acute attack, especially in cases of allergic asthma. This substance is known as sodium cromoglycate and is available both in powder and solution form, which can be inhaled regularly to prevent attacks. This would fail in case an allergic process has started to cascade. Encouraging results are seen in children with allergic symptoms and in people who suffer from exercise-induced asthma. In fact, this chemical is now available in a standard eyedrop preparation which gives good results in cases of allergic conjunctivitis.

This compound is extremely safe and useful. The only problem that is encountered by some people is bronchoconstriction on inhaling sodium cromoglycate. This can be prevented by a bronchodilator or an inhaled corticosteroid. Sodium cromoglycate works on an average for four to six hours, after which it is broken down by the body. Thus one would require four inhalations in a day. This powder is available in capsule form, which is put in a small apparatus called the 'spinhaler'. The capsule is ruptured, the powder released and is inhaled.

All in all, this is a good and safe preventive medicine to be taken on a regular basis, especially during the months of allergy but it has no role in managing an acute attack or in people who do not have allergic asthma.

Bronchodilators

As the most distressing symptom is caused by narrowing or constriction of the airways, relief is felt when we dilate or rather, cause counter-constriction through medication. One needs to understand this in a

Asthmatics should avoid pain-killers, like Aspirin and Ibuprofen. These medicines could precipitate an asthmatic attack.

Pain-killers block inflammatory substances called prostaglandins, thereby precipitating acute attacks of asthma.

Acetoaminophen or Paracetamol is a medicine which can be taken for pain relief by asthmatics.

little detailed fashion. The muscle tone of the bronchial passages is controlled by:

- Sympathetic nervous system which causes bronchodilatation.
- Vagus nerve which causes constriction of the passages.

Thus, all medicines, which work like the sympathetic nerve, cause bronchodilatation and are thus, as a group, called bronchodilators. Another group called anticholinergic drugs or vagomimetic (antivagus nerve action) can also prevent bronchoconstriction.

Drugs which work on the sympathetic nerve are the sympathomimetic medicines which are the most popular and widely used bronchodilators. Herbal concoctions used for controlling cough had Ephedrine which is used in modern medicine till date. Newer, safer and more effective drugs are now in the market and are of great use. These work very well during attacks and great relief is provided to an asthmatic if given in the right dosage schedule. The discovery of adrenaline was a landmark though the route through which it is given is not a very convenient one. Many newer products have since invaded the market. One common problem faced with this medicine group is the trembling of the hands and at times, quickening of the heart rate. These cause a lot of uneasiness but are harmless — the patient notices these only for the first week or two.

Anticholinergics

There are medicines which have been in use for some time now. In an inhaled form, these work well and have almost no side effects. Iratropium bromide is underused and its full potential has neither been realised nor understood.

Xanthine derivatives

Xanthine derivatives, especially theophylline, is a potent and good bronchodilator. It works directly on the smooth muscles of the bronchial passage, thereby getting rid of bronchial constriction. This product is available in tablet form and as a suppository. The drug is of immense help in treating severe bronchospasms in an OPD or hospital setup where an intravenous injection or slow drip of a xanthine derivative is given. In most cases, it works like magic. At times, these can be mixed with an intravenous corticosteroid to obtain better and faster results.

Corticosteroids

To use or not to use — that is the question. Lots of debates and lots of badly managed patients by quacks, godmen and lay people tell the dismal story of corticosteroid abuse. There is no denying the fact that corticosteroids are among the most potent of bronchodilators available. They have been in vogue for decades and in India, this assumes great importance. All wonder powders, *bhasmas* (burnt ash) and sure-shot therapies available, should be carefully tested for the presence of corticosteroids. People take these and obtain quick and complete recovery from asthma, but, they soon report with puffiness of the face, thinning of the legs, etc. which indicate the side effects of corticosteroids. Also the word 'steroid' evokes fear in many because the drugs are associated with images of beefy, muscle-bound body-builders, masculinised women, or Olympic cheats who died young or of obese moonfaced patients.

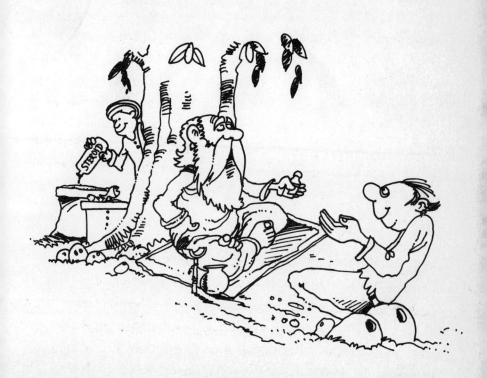

Anything good if misused or used indiscriminately would have grave effects and so does it happen with corticosteroid tablets. These should be taken once in the morning after meals, so as to avoid disturbing the pituitary gland–adrenal gland axis. Looking at the long list of its serious side effects, it is best to use the medicine only if all other medicines have failed. It is most intelligent to use all other drugs before we think of any steroid therapy. Despite all this care, there is a certain percentage of people who would not respond to anything else — for them only corticosteroids could help save life. In such cases, a careful minimum dosage schedule monitored regularly and tapered or stopped when not required would be an intelligent regime.

Aerosols and intramuscular injections are also available. Aerosols are easy to carry and effective but could cause throat irritation, dryness of throat, hoarseness of voice or rarely, fungal infection of the mouth or gums. Still, it is a great medicine if used intelligently and as a last resort. Now you might be wondering as to why so much caution needs to be observed in the use of corticosteroids! Let's enumerate the side effects so that the mystery gets solved:

- It is a catabolic drug, i.e. it helps in the breakdown of proteins causing atrophy of the skin with thining of the skin; the bones become brittle and fracture easily; the backbone collapses; the patient's face swells up and the legs become thin.
- It could precipitate or unmask high blood pressure.
- It could cause diabetes mellitus.
- It may lead to gastritis and gastric ulceration.
- It may upset the body's production of cortisone, proving catastrophic for the patient.

The long list is not to scare the patients but to educate them about the intelligent usage of steroids in asthmatics (who do not respond to other medicines).

CHAPTER SEVEN

Drug delivery system

Often physicians are asked this question: 'Don't you think the use of an inhaler makes you get hooked on to it?' The answer is a definite 'no'. Let me first explain the different modes of the drug delivery system.

Aerosols or inhalers usually propel a drug at a great speed. The particle size is usually very small and the medicine is pushed into the respiratory system along with the inhaled air to reach the bronchial tree and work on the muscles. Aerosols are available freely and are very handy.

While swallowing or injecting excess-steroids into one's body is dangerous, the doses of inhaled steroids prescribed in modern asthma inhalers are too small to have adverse effects. It is usually recommended that

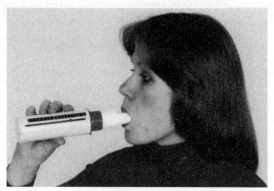
Check your lung capacity

these drugs be taken once or twice a day through an inhaler or a puffer. Learning the proper technique of using the inhaler is vital to ensure that one inhales the right dose of drug correctly into the airways.

It is important to always wash one's mouth with water after inhalation to make certain that any steroid particles, left in the mouth and throat, are not swallowed.

If taken in the right way, inhaled steroids prove most effective in minimising the frequency and severity of asthma attacks.

If an attack occurs despite taking one's preventive medication regularly, a reliever medication is prescribed. A common reliever drug in use worldwide is Salbutamol, but there are several in the market today available in the form of inhalers that deliver a measured dose of the drug. These medications exert their effects by relieving the spasm in the bronchial muscles and widening the air tubes, thus allowing more air to flow into and out of the lungs.

Aerosol corticosteroid preparations are widely used, but I would recommend the use of aerosol bronchodilator first. The aerosol works very fast and can be taken on an S.O.S. basis, i.e. if and when required. One metered dose is a standard dose and instructions about dosage need to be followed strictly.

Rotahalers are small, plastic apparatuses in which one could insert a powder-filled capsule. Once the capsule is pushed in, you twist the upper part of the rotahaler. This breaks the rotacap and the powder is released. It is then sucked in with the inhaled air and it starts to work. The benefit of this mode of treatment is its light weight and it is also fairly inexpensive. The only drawback is that certain people

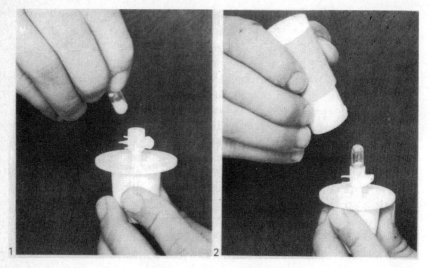

Method of Loading a Spinhaler

find the powder entering the throat, a little irritating. Some patients complain of a mild cough after the use of a rotahaler.

Nebulisers are possibly the most sophisticated of the entire lot of gizmos for drug delivery. In this, a solution is nebulised and a fine spray is inhaled through a face mask. It is a much more effective delivery system as compared to a rotahaler/inhaler. The flip side is

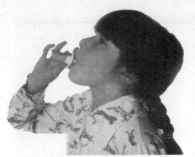

Using an Intal Spinhaler

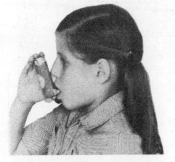

Using a Bronchodilator

that it is a more expensive and bulky apparatus. Also, the entire process of nebulisation could take 10 to 20 minutes. Yet, it remains the physician's favoured delivery system.

The plus point of aerosol therapy is that the dose of the medicine used is very low. Also, it does not enter the blood and thus, there are hardly any systemic side affects. Also, it acts very fast and can be taken by the patient himself in acute attacks or just prior to an acute attack.

CHAPTER EIGHT

Status asthmaticus and its management

Acute attacks of asthma are very distressing. If an acute asthmatic episode lasts more than 12 hours, it is termed *'status asthmaticus'*. Status asthmaticus is a medical emergency and the patient should be admitted to a proper care centre. The problem in such cases is that exhalation becomes more and more difficult. Most of the times, inhaled aerosols do not seem to work because these cannot reach the constricted airways. Coupled with muscular exertion, the panic reaction and the increasing breathlessness make this a critical condition. Usually most patients would respond to an intravenous injection of a xanthine derivative and a corticosteroid. If this does not seem to work, a continuous intravenous medication in the form of a bronchodilator and a corticosteroid is advisable. If the patient still does not respond, rarely one has to intubate the patient and put the patient on a respirator. This means introducing a catheter into the trachea through the throat and connecting it to a machine which takes on the role of the lungs. Once the patient is out of status asthmaticus, the tube can be withdrawn.

'Where there is no cure, there are a hundred cures', goes an old adage and how right its sounds in this context. People resort to some fish treatment, acupuncture and also surgeries. All in all, the managememt of asthma is good, but a cure for asthma is still a puzzle.

Action plan

An important aspect of asthma management these days is to have a written Asthma Action Plan, a copy of which should be kept with the patient or with the parents and teacher if the patient is a child. The purpose of such a written plan is to educate the person about asthma so that he or she knows why the different medications are taken, how they should be taken and when.

The 'when' aspect is most important so that he/she does not neglect to take the preventive medication regularly, and that he/she knows what symptoms indicate that it is time to take a dose of the reliever medication.

Of course, having a plan and buying the correct medications prescribed by the physician are only part of the solution.

Far too many people with asthma forget to take their reliever puff when they leave home or have the puff in their pocket or handbag but feel embarrassed to take it out and resist using it even when they feel tightness in the chest.

Just one more thing: *Don't forget to take your medications.*

CHAPTER NINE

Antigens that cause allergy

Plant origin

- Cotton
- Flour/bran
- Wood dust
- Pollen
- Moulds
- Coffee and cocoa beans

Animial origin

- Domesticated animals
- Birds and poultry
- Furs of animals
- Insects
- Mites in dust

Chemicals

- Dust/aerosols
- Petroleum products
- Metals like nickel, platinum

Human origin

- Hair
- Hairwigs

Indicators for specfic allergies

- *Hair dye allergy:*
  (a) Allergy or itching of the scalp within one or two days of using hair dye.

(b) Itching on the neck and behind the ears.

- *Food allergy:*
  - Vomiting each time one has a particular food item.
  - Rash on the lips or inside the mouth every time you eat that particular food item.
  - Is there stomach ache or loose motions on eating a particular thing?

If the answer to any of the above three questions is 'yes', then you have a food-induced allergy.

Common food items causing allergy are:

- Fruits like:

  Bananas
  Grapefruits
  Oranges
  Apples

- Vegetables like:

  Garlic
  Onions
  Radish

- High protein
  sources:

  Soyabeans
  Mushrooms
  Eggs

- Nuts like: Cashewnuts

- Fish

- Wheat

All these allergies can be managed by avoiding the above-mentioned food items but the problem arises when milk allergy (other than mother's milk), is seen in about three to five per thousand children. The child tends to suffer from abdominal pain and at times vomiting or loose motions. When skin allergy and eczematous-like diagnoses are seen, avoid milk for some time and then reintroduce it. If symptoms return or persist, then diagnosis stands confirmed. Management is to withdraw animal source milk and start on soya milk (derived from soyabeans).

Hay fever

How often have you heard the term 'hay fever'? Very often, you must admit, though most of the times the speaker is not sure as to what hay fever means. This is a condition caused by allergy to grass pollen, which could cause itching followed by a stuffy feeling in the nose. One could feel the whole head, especially the forehead, congested. Certain others would without a warning start to sneeze repeatedly and, at times violently, followed by a running nose. The allergy does not spare the eyes which too become itchy, red, watery and at times, puffy. Often there is a funny, itchy sensation in the palate. Many hay fever patients complain of a blocked sensation in the ears and that their own voice sounds like an echo. This is the entire spectrum of hay fever. This set of symptoms would appear every year or at times twice a year at the same time of the year because pollen of a plant is released into the atmosphere during a particular weather.

The close association between hay fever and asthma shows that these are different sides to the same coin. People suffering from hay fever could have bouts of cough with wheezing. At the same time, people with bronchial asthma may possibly show symptoms of hay fever in the initial stage. Thus, the close relationship between the two has been established.

The management broadly falls under diagnosis of the 'culprit' pollen and treatment with antihistamines and, at times, nasal aerosols of corticosteroids. If the condition is not managed properly, it could cause a disease of the nasal mucosa, resulting in nasal polyp formation and, at times, chronic sinusitis.

Managing asthma is not difficult if we make the effort to understand our condition, educate ourselves about our medications, and ask our physician to write out a practical Action Plan to follow.

Wrap up

Looking at the extent of allergic manifestations in our population, managing the same at each possible level becomes imperative. Cleaning up our immediate vicinity and our good earth should be our first priority. Patient education and early treatment would be equally important. Last but not least, research and newer forms of treatment modes should be encouraged. The indomitable human can and will achieve success. May God bless humans!

Questions on first visit

It is always good to be prepared before you visit your doctor. The following questions your doctor may ask when you visit him or her for the first time.

- Any history of sneezing spells, when weather changes   Yes/No

- Any history of running nose   Yes/No

- History of cough at each weather change   Yes/No

- History of breathlessness   Yes/No

- Any family history of asthma   Yes/No

- Any history of eczema during childhood   Yes/No

- Any history of allergic eye condition   Yes/No

- Any history of residing in high pollen areas   Yes/No

- How polluted is your city?   Clean/polluted/very polluted